How To Make Homemade Face Mask and Homemade Hand Sanitizer

A Step-by-Step Guide to Making Face Mask and Hand Sanitizer To Protect You Against Infectious Diseases Caused By Viruses And Bacteria

JAMEKA WATKINS

ISBN: 9798636115809

CONTENTS

Introduction

1 PART I: KNOW YOUR HAND SANITIZER Page 1

Why Hand Sanitizer NOW? Page 2

Why Home-Made? Page 5

What are the critical ingredients? Page 7

Other essential but non-critical ingredients Page 11

2 PART II: YOUR HAND SANITIZER RECIPES Page 17

Recipes with Alcohol as the main critical ingredient Page 18

Recipes with Witch Hazel as the main critical ingredient Page 23

Combo Recipes Page 31

Mild and Miscellaneous recipes Page 36

WHO & CDC Recommended formulation Page 40

3 PART III: TIPS & FAQS Page 47

Tips Page 48

FAQs Page 53

4 FACE MASK Page 56

Mask Classificaion Page 58

Respiratory Protection Page 61

The different types of masks Page 61

How to chose my respiratory mask? Page 63

What is the Corona Virus? Page 64

Homemade mask DIY   Page 71

Homemade Face mask an example of DIY   Page 77

Conclusion   Page 83

INTRODUCTION

"First came the SARS, I thought then that it was the Far East and thus it didn't concern me.

Then came the MERS that started from the Middle East. I thought that it was still East – though in the Middle, and thus it still didn't concern me.

And NOW, there is COVID-19, which started from South East, spread so fast in all directions, and then right in the West where I am.

I now realize that it concerned ME - right from the start. Before this realization, I treated it just horror news... from far off lands... aware but unperturbed.

But NOW, resting on my hospital bed, I realize that if I got concerned about it early enough, I would have kept a Hand Sanitizer. But, even with MONEY, the URGENCY OF NOW means that it cannot be found in the shops... and thus can't keep my family and loved ones safe.

Maybe if I were conscious enough, and I had appreciated the magnitude and risk of this group of infectious viruses, I would have learned to make my own hand sanitizer. I wouldn't be hopelessly in bed. My loved ones wouldn't be now quarantined. And probably, I would have saved others.

I would have saved my family. And my family would have kept my neighbors. And my neighbors would have saved my community. And my community would have saved my nation. And my nation would have saved the world.

I deeply regret my ignorance."

--- Echoes from the mind of a Corona Virus victim.

Yes, and as the Far East sages once said, "If you are planning for a season, plant rice; if you are planning for a decade, plant trees; but if you are planning for a lifetime, educate people." I have decided to plan for a lifetime... to educate people. And this book is my piece of education that I am providing you. I don't want you to regret it later.

We surely don't know what will come after the Corona Virus. But, if all of us learn how to make a Hand Sanitizer, we wouldn't wait for the 'demons' hiding within these viruses to come and rob the lives of our loved ones. We would secure their lives and their future. Yet, this is no miracle. There is no charm in it. Simple knowledge of how to make one of the most critical hygiene tools – the Hand Sanitizer, is all one needs. I don't mean that hand sanitizer is the panacea for all infections, but it can play its active role in mitigating the risks.

Don't become a victim of ignorance. Don't spare avenues for regrets. Secure yourself, family, and loved ones. Learn how to make Hand Sanitizer… right in your house.

Let me show you HOW!

PART I: KNOW YOUR HAND SANITIZER

Sometimes, something can be so familiar such that we overlook its most important details. Hand sanitizer is one such item.

Do you really know your hand sanitizer?

This so obvious question can, at times strike our nerves. One may easily be tempted to say "of course, yes." Yet, when it comes to explaining simple details such as its core ingredients, the main functions of each of these core ingredients, and the mix ratio - that becomes another chemistry lesson to crack… and a hard one.

And yet, you ought to really know your hand sanitizer well. In critical moments like this one that we are living in… where one infectious epidemic subsides, only to beckon the next one… you cannot afford to take such easy questions for granted.

It is for this reason that I have decided to provide you with the basic 101 info about your hand sanitizer. You never know, this could be all you need to protect your life and that of your loved ones from the storm of an epidemic.

Why Hand Sanitizer NOW?

Hands serve important functions in our lives. They are the most preferred way of greetings, especially with face-to-face encounters.

The food we eat requires the use of hands. Even if you are using forks, spoons, and serviettes, that doesn't stop germs on the hands from falling into that food on the plate or saucer. Maybe, you can only guarantee this by wearing hand gloves. But, what would you be using to wear the hand gloves? Robots? No, still your hands or someone else's hands.

We also use hands when in the lavatories and washrooms. We hardly wear gloves before going to such places. Meaning? We often run the risk of carrying germs from the washrooms and lavatories.

So, what is the best way to keep off germs? Hand sanitizer!

We are so accustomed to handing sanitizers that they have become some kind of little shrines where we pay some sort of ritual. Have you ever asked yourself, "What does this sanitizer contain?" and, "How does it really work?" and more importantly, "Can I make it?"

You better have answers to these questions at your fingertips.

Why hand sanitizer? The simple answer is: TO KILL GERMS!

Yet, this answer, however accurate it is, remains veiled. Not that it is not adequate, but, while it answers the 'Why?' it doesn't answer the 'What?' and the 'How?' And even if it somehow answers the 'Why?' it doesn't yet answer, the 'Why NOW?'

So, Why Hand Sanitizer NOW?

NOW! This is extremely urgent. I guess you've heard of CORONA VIRUS. Yes, that virus, which is spreading faster than wildfire. I guess you've already heard of SARS (Severe Acute Respiratory Syndrome), MERS (Middle-East Acute Respiratory Syndrome), and of late COVID-19 (SARS 2).

Why NOW? Yes, the clue rests in how countries and people have handled the Corona Virus. In its aftermath, it hasn't spared even the wealthiest of nations. Both the rich and the poor have certain bad hygiene habits that make them susceptible to such infections. One such bad hygienic habit is not having a hand sanitizer always within your reach.

The rapid spread SARS-COV-2 virus that causes COVID-19 syndrome makes NOW bolder and pronounced than ever before. The thousands of infections and the hundreds of deaths a day make it a mimic of global Armageddon. Eventually, this will subside, but we are still yet to know what this vampire will mutate into in its next incarnation.

The NOW desperation

When Coronavirus broke up in China, one of those things that ran scarce is the hand sanitizer. In Wuhan, the epicenter of this virus-stricken country, people rushed to the shops and bought all the much that they could of hand sanitizers.

The biggest desperation is when you have money to buy a life-saving remedy, yet it is not available. So much desperation when you thought that having money in your account could save you against emergencies only to realize that, in some cases, money becomes worthless... and that something that used to be cheaply available has become much more scarce than gold. Yet, you can live without gold, but not without health.

It is such desperation when you and your loved ones are suffering simply because something so cheap that almost everyone could afford without a sweat is no longer available. You hear deaths roaming in your town, deaths menacing in your community, and deaths shouting in your neighborhoods — and its psychological stench passing right through your nose, yet, you can do nothing.

It is such desperation when you realize that that cheap substance is also very easy to make... but, because you took it for granted due to its cheap availability, you never learned how to make it.

And the NOW PANIC BUYING

In the early aftermath of COVID-19, Panic triggered PANIC BUYING, which induced hyper-demand. And this HYPER DEMAND created hoarding and shortages. The result was that PEOPLE HAD MONEY BUT NO HAND SANITIZERS.

Yes, WHEN CORONA VIRUS STRIKES YOUR AREA, NOT EVEN YOUR MONEY CAN SAVE YOU! You may have the money, but miss on the Hand Sanitizer!

HAVE MONEY BUT NO HAND SANITIZERS in the shops? What can you do?

The simple answer is that YOU HAVE TO MAKE YOUR OWN Hand Sanitizer.

And it is for this reason that I have decided to write this book. Yes, to save you from the vagaries of PANIC BUYING. To save you from that helpless situation whereby you desperately need a hand sanitizer, but it is neither in the shops nor stores and there is nothing your money can do about it.

Make your own!

And in this book, we are going to show you HOW!

Why Home-Made?

Why NOT?

Anyway, we've already hinted as to why you need to have Home-made Hand Sanitizer. The main reason is that, whenever there is an epidemic, people rush to buy. Before factories ramp up production to meet the spike in demand, the supermarket shelves are already empty. But, can factories ramp up production when workers are advised to stay at home during the epidemic?

Yet, like astute businesspeople, suppliers would be hesitant to suddenly ramp up production unless they study the demand pattern. They don't want to risk overproduction. And also, stores don't want to risk overstocking. In the meanwhile, scarcity is biting while the epidemic is mauling people down by their thousands.

To avoid being stuck between the devil that is the epidemic and the wall that is scarcity, you have to think well in advance. You have to equip yourself. And like a shrewd prepper, you have to equip yourself with the skills of how to make it yourself… so that the only remaining task is to keep the ingredients within reach.

If you can't find it, make it!
Well, necessity is the mother of invention. As per the law of demand and supply, the more demand outstrips supply, the more the price skyrockets. Why not reap from your entrepreneurial spirit? Anyway, we are not here to discuss as to how you can turn into an overnight millionaire by taking advantage of this ocean-gap scarcity, but, rather, we are here to discuss the compelling health and safety reasons as to why you must learn how to make your own Sanitizer – right at home!

The EXTRA benefits!
Other than avoiding being caught between the wall of scarcity and the daredevil of epidemics, there quite a great number of benefits that you can gain:

- Ability to save your life and that of others – in a difficult situation such as that where there is an outbreak of Corona Virus or such related epidemics, being able to make your own hand sanitizer when there no such left in the stores means saving lives by protecting them against infections.

- A new skill – learning to make your own hand sanitizer is actually gaining an industrial skill. This skill can become important during prepping and survival in difficult conditions.

- More affordable solution during periods of hyper-demand – under normal circumstances, manufactured hand sanitizers are relatively cheap compared to home-made ones. However, when there is an epidemic outbreak, there is a spike in demand for the manufactured ones such that the price skyrockets making home-made sanitizers more economical, especially if you can brew your own alcohol.

- Opportunity to make money – you can make money while saving lives during an epidemic when manufactured hand sanitizers run dry on the shop shelves.

Is it safe?

Yes! PROPERLY HOME-MADE hand sanitizer is safe to use. However, just as pharmaceutically-made hand sanitizers, ensure that the ingredients are of the right quality, devices used are clean and toxin-free, and you make the right mix proportions. And this is why I am here to show you HOW!

What are the critical ingredients?

Critical ingredients are those ingredients without which you cannot even talk of hand sanitizer. The critical ingredients fall into two main categories:

1.   Disinfectants

2.   Moisturizers

The Disinfectants
The disinfectants are those ingredients that are directly responsible for killing the germs. The four most commonly used disinfectants for home-made hand sanitizers are:

1.   Alcohol

2.   Hydrogen Peroxide

3.   Witch Hazel

4.   Vinegar

Alcohol
Alcohol is the most crucial ingredient in the hand sanitizer. Alcohol has been used for ages as a disinfectant on wounds. So, it naturally found its place in hand sanitizers.

What type of alcohol is recommended?
There are two main types of alcohol that you should use:

- Isopropyl alcohol (rubbing alcohol)

- Ethanol (grain alcohol)

What type of alcohol should I not use?
You should not use Butanol, Methanol, and such other types of alcohol as they are toxic.

What is the recommended alcohol volume?
It is recommended that the final product (that is, hand sanitizer) should have an alcohol content of at least 60%. Since alcohol content should be 2/3 of the final product, then it means that the volume of alcohol in terms of

proofs should be at least 91%.

What is the primary function of alcohol?
Alcohol serves three primary functions:

- Disinfectant – as a disinfectant, alcohol kills germs that are present.

- Solvent – as a solvent, alcohol helps to dissolve other ingredients into a soluble form.

- Preservative – with alcohol, your sanitizer can be kept for months, and it will be improved with the addition of hydrogen peroxide.

Alcohol alternatives/substitutes
Just in case alcohol is not available within your locality or for some other reasons, the following are its main alternatives:

1. Witch Hazel

2. Hydrogen Peroxide

3. Vinegar

4. Bleach

Witch Hazel is the best alternative in case you are avoiding alcohol due to your skin sensitivity – especially if your skin is ultra-dry.

Hydrogen peroxide
Hydrogen Peroxide is a naturally occurring compound that is commonly found in rainwater and snow. Hydrogen Peroxide is widely known as Oxygen Water since it is water with an extra oxygen molecule (i.e., $H2O + O = H2O2$).

Hydrogen Peroxide comes in various grades, depending on its targeted usage. The 3% pharmaceutical grade is the one recommended for hand sanitizers.

Vinegar

Vinegar is a mild antibacterial agent. Nonetheless, it is claimed to kill 99% of bacteria. The most significant advantage of vinegar is that it is cheaply available. Another significant advantage is that, since it is edible, non-toxic, and non-pollutant, it can be used to disinfect fresh fruits and vegetables thus making sure that you ingest bacteria-free food.

When it comes to hand sanitizer, the most commonly used or recommended vinegar is 5% white vinegar.

You can use vinegar either on its own as a hand sanitizer, or you can blend it with essential oils to obfuscate the strong smell. However, it takes just a few minutes for your hands to become odor-free, even without the need for fragrance.

In case you urgently need to make a hand sanitizer but don't have alcohol or hydrogen peroxide available, vinegar serves as a good alternative.

Bleach

Bleach is mainly used to disinfect utensils before using them to make your hand sanitizer. Generally, it is not mixed with other ingredients in the formulation of hand sanitizer.

Bleach is often used when hydrogen peroxide is not available to disinfect the utensils.

Skin Moisturizers

While disinfectants kill germs, most of them are not soft on your skin. Most of them, especially alcohol and hydrogen peroxide, leave your skin dry and, at times, irritated.

To keep your skin moist, you should need to have skin moisturizer as part of the essential ingredients. This is extremely important because dry skin easily cracks and thus creating avenues for new infections that cannot be stopped by the alcohol that has already evaporated.

The following are some of the most commonly used skin moisturizers when it comes to home-made hand sanitizers:

1.   Aloe Vera

2.   Vitamin E oil

3.   Glycerin

4.   Essential oil moisturizers – e.g., Tea Tree Oil

Aloe Vera
Aloe Vera is probably the most widely used herb when it comes to the cosmetic and pharmaceutical industries. This is due to its diverse therapeutic properties.

Why Aloe Vera?
As we have indicated, Aloe Vera is extremely versatile when it comes to therapeutic properties. This makes it serve both internal and external usage.

- Nonetheless, the following are the fundamental properties that make it useful as an essential ingredient in the hand sanitizer:

- Antimicrobial properties – Aloe Vera kills a wide array of bacteria. When mixed with alcohol, this boosts the efficacy of the resultant product.

- Healing properties – Aloe Vera helps to heal small wounds. This is more important knowing that dry skin (as a result of alcohol) is more susceptible to cracks.

- Anti-inflammation properties – this is the main reason why it is used in combination with alcohol. Aloe Vera alleviates irritation due to dry skin.

- Moisturizer – the skin protective properties in Aloe Vera makes it act as a veneer against rapid evaporation.

Aloe Vera alternatives
In case you cannot find Aloe Vera within your locality, or you are allergic to it, then you would need to use its options.

The following are the most commonly used Aloe Vera alternatives:

1.   Glycerin
2.   Vitamin E oil
3.   Tea Tree oil
4.   Lavender

Other essential but non-critical ingredients

Other than disinfectants and moisturizers, you can optionally add more ingredients to make your hand sanitizer much better.

The following are the critical properties that such essential but non-critical ingredients can add to your home-made hand sanitizer:

- Anti-inflammation

- Skin toning

- Fragrance

Some ingredients can have several of these properties plus more. For example, while we considered Aloe Vera as an essential moisturizer, it does also possess anti-inflammation and skin toning properties. What it doesn't have is the admirable fragrance.

The following are the key properties of the critical but non-critical ingredients that you can optionally add to your home-made hand sanitizer:

1. Essential Oils

2. Glycerin

Essential Oils
Essential oils are naturally occurring aromatic found in plant flowers, seeds, barks, stems, roots, and other plant parts. They are highly volatile as they can easily change from liquid to gaseous state.

Essential oils are widely used for skin care. This is the first reason as to why they are part of the ingredients in most hand sanitizers – to take care of the skin.

The following are the most widely used application of essential oils for skincare:

1. Anti-wrinkles

2. Anti-aging

3.   Acne

Essential oils for wrinkles:

1.   Geranium Essential Oil.

2.   Tea Tree Essential Oil.

3.   Lavender Essential Oil.

4.   Neroli Essential Oil.

5.   Myrrh Essential Oil.

6.   Frankincense Essential Oil.

7.   Patchouli Essential Oil.

8.   Neroli Essential Oil.

Anti-aging Essential oils:

1.   Coconut Oil.

2.   Carrot Seed Oil.

3.   Geranium Oil.

4.   Argan Oil.

5.   Sweet Almond Oil.

6.   Avocado Oil.

7.   Apricot Kernel Oil.

8.   Rosehip Seed Oil.

Essential oils for acne and pimples:

Juniper Berry.

Tea Tree.

Clary Sage.

Lavender.

Essential oils are very diverse. Some of the functions of essential oils include:

- Purifiers-cinnamon, eucalyptus, lavender, peppermint, thyme, rosemary, clove

- Nourishers – Vitamin E essential oil

- Germ destroyers – Tea tree oil, lavender

- Anti-inflammation and skin-soothing – Tea Tree Oil, Frankincense Essential Oil, lavender.

- Moisturizer – Vitamin E Oil

- Skin toner - Geranium essential oil,

- Fragrance – Lavender, peppermint, Ylang Ylang

Special mentions

Just as "some animals are more equal than others," so it is that "some essential oils are more equal than others." This compels us to have a special mention of this particular kind of essential oils:

Tea Tree Oil

Tea Tree Oil is probably the most important of all essential oils when it comes to hand sanitizer. This is because it has antiviral, antifungal, antimicrobial, antibacterial, and antiseptic properties.

Thus, Tea Tree Oil is a disinfectant in its own right. Though, it is not as potent as alcohol or hydrogen peroxide.

Lavender

When it comes to fragrance, Lavender is the most widely used essential oil. However, it is not just a fragrance. Its sweet smell can easily disguise its potent antiviral and antibacterial properties.

Lemongrass Oil

Lemongrass is not as commonly used as Tea Tree Oil and Lavender.

However, when you don't have the two, it can be a fair substitute.

Glycerin

Glycerin is popularly known for its dense thickness that is colorless, odorless, and sweet-tasting. It is a byproduct of the soap making process. Plant glycerin is composed of sugar and organic alcohol compound. There is also animal glycerin. It is common to have a blend of both plant and animal glycerin.

Glycerin has been widely used in the hair and beauty products for ages. A good number of hair and beauty products do have glycerin.

When it comes to hand sanitizer, glycerin plays the following role:

- Anti-aging – glycerin helps to keep your skin wrinkle-free. This makes you look younger and vibrant.

- Moisturizer – as a complement or alternative to Aloe Vera, glycerin works as a moisturizer. This makes it an excellent option for those who are allergic to Aloe Vera.

- Emollient – glycerin acts as an emollient by not only moisturizing the skin but also softening it. Softening the skin prevents cracking, which brings irritation and susceptibility to infections. Thus, glycerin guards against itching and flaking, the common side-effects of alcohol disinfectant in the sanitizer.

- Skin toner – soothes and smoothens dry skin.

- Cleanser – glycerin is commonly used as an ingredient in facial scrubs due to its cleansing properties. It cleanses the skin pores, thus removing stuck toxins, thus opening up the pores.

- Sunscreen – glycerin can protect your skin from destructive ultra-violet rays.

- Antifungal – Glycerin has antifungal properties that can help you heal from fungal infections. It is reasonably effective in alleviating psoriasis and eczema.
- Exfoliator – glycerin acts as a soft exfoliator. It achieves this by breaking down the protein fiber in dead skin cells and thus removes these unconscious elements from the skin, leaving it clear and healthy.

Vitamin E Oil

When it comes to skin moisturizing and softening effect, Vitamin E oil is one of the most recognized emollients. This oil is widely used in skin and hair products.

Apart from making your hand feel soft, Vitamin E Oil keeps the hand sanitizer fresh.

Want pure natural ingredients?

Yes, you can have them. And yes, you use them. And still, yes, you can make them!

Pure natural ingredients are those ingredients that are fully natural without the addition of synthetic chemicals. This means that even the alcohol used should be obtained from natural sources, fermented, and distilled through the natural process.

Pure natural ingredients for your hand sanitizer

Most of the components that we have discussed can be obtained in their pure natural form. Thus, if you want to use pure natural ingredients, simply get them and apply them in your recipes just as the synthetic ingredients, for so long as you achieve the same concentration level.

What we won't be discussing

Unless you live on farmlands where you can grow your own corn or other plant sources of alcohol for the brewing process, then you will need to buy ready-made natural (grain) alcohol (ethanol), which is also commonly used as biofuel.

In this book, I assume that you can easily access this natural alcohol. So, we won't be discussing the brewing and distillation process. The same is the case with Aloe Vera and essential oils. And just like alcohol, I won't be discussing how to extract Aloe Vera from Aloe Vera plant and make Aloe Vera gel. I won't also be talking about how to extract essential oils. There are plenty of materials online and other dedicated books on the topic that you can refer to if you want to make the extracts yourself.

What I expect from you
I assume that you have access to natural alcohol of at least 91% volume, and you also have access to natural extracts of Aloe Vera and essential oils.

Water!
Water is important. Water is essential for moisturizing and also for diluting some of the concentrated ingredients.

While not all recipes will need water, those recipes that need water must be given careful consideration.

Type of water

In case you need water for your hand sanitizer, it should have the following qualities:

- Clean – free from visible impurities

- Distilled (or boiled)

- Sterilized

PART II: YOUR HAND SANITIZER RECIPES

Now that you understand the core ingredients of your hand sanitizer and the critical functions of each component, the next logical step is to satisfy your hunger for skills… that is, how to make your own.

Hunger no more. Here I unveil the 22 simple recipes that you can use to make your own home-made hand sanitizer.

Each recipe means that you are a step ahead of the pandemic storm. And each recipe suggests that you, your family, and loved ones have a strong shield against infections.

Be forearmed. Be prepared. Prevention is better than cure.

Recipes with Alcohol as the main critical ingredient

You can either use Ethanol or Isopropyl alcohol. If you are using ethanol, make sure that it is at least 97% volume. If you are using Isopropyl alcohol, make sure that it is at least 99% volume. This will make your hand sanitizer effective even during an epidemic. You never know where and whom an epidemic strikes… it could be you. So protect yourself before it strikes by having the right germ-killing concentrations.

Recipe 1 – Spray-based hand sanitizer with alcohol and Aloe Vera as active ingredients

Primary ingredients: Alcohol and Aloe Vera

Tools & Equipment

- Bowl

- Spoon

- Funnel

- Bottle with a pump dispenser

Ingredients

- 2/3 cup of 99% alcohol (ethanol or isopropyl)

- 1/3 cup of Aloe Vera

- 10 drops of your preferred essential oil (optional)

Instructions

1. Mix all the ingredients.

2. Whisk the ingredients to achieve a uniform texture.

3. Using the funnel, carefully pour the mixed ingredients into the bottle and screw up the bottle top to tighten.

4. Set for about 30 minutes and then use it when needed.

Advisory notes

You can use the product immediately after pouring it into the bottle. However, giving time for the mixture to set ensures that the chemical mix is optimized. Also, penetrating and killing spores takes some time. WHO recommends at least 72 hours, guaranteeing that spores are done away with.

Recipe 2 – Squirt-based hand sanitizer with Alcohol and Aloe Vera as primary ingredients

Primary ingredients: Alcohol and Aloe Vera

Tools & Equipment

- Small bowl

- Spoon

- Funnel

- Squirt bottle

Ingredients

- 3 ounces of 99% alcohol (ethanol or isopropyl)

- 1 ounce of Aloe Vera gel

- ¼ teaspoon of Vitamin E Oil

- a combination of essential oil (optional)

Combination of essential oils:

- 30 drops of tea tree oil

- 8 drops of lavender essential oil

Instructions

1. Drop all the essential oils into a small bowl and mix by swirling

2. Pour alcohol into the essential oils mix and swirl further

3.   Add Aloe Vera into the mix and whisk the ingredients to achieve a uniform texture.

4.   Put the mixture into the squirt bottle and tighten the top

5.   Set for about 30 minutes and then use it when needed.

Advisory notes
Use a colored bottle to avoid intense light interfering with the essential oils in the hand sanitizer. If you prefer a spray instead of a gel, you can substitute Aloe Vera with Witch Hazel.

Recipe 3 – Squeezable hand sanitizer with Alcohol and Aloe Vera as primary ingredients

Primary ingredients: Alcohol and Aloe
Vera Tools & Equipment

- Small bowl

- Spoon

- Squeezable bottle

Ingredients

- 1 tablespoon of 99% alcohol (ethanol or isopropyl)

- 3 tablespoon of Aloe Vera gel

- a combination of essential oil (optional)

Combination of essential oils:

- 1 teaspoon of Vitamin E Oil

- 2 drops of tea tree oil

- 3 drops of purifier essential oil (e.g., eucalyptus, peppermint, cinnamon, thyme, lavender, clove, or rosemary)

Instructions

1.   Drop all the essential oils into a small bowl and mix by swirling

2.   Pour alcohol into the essential oils mix and swirl further

3.   Add Aloe Vera into the mix and whisk the ingredients to achieve a uniform texture.

4.   Put the mixture into the squeezable bottle and tighten thc top

5.   Set for about 30 minutes and then use it when needed.

Advisory notes
Use a colored bottle to avoid intense light interfering with the essential oils in the hand sanitizer. If you want a spray instead of a gel, you can substitute Aloe Vera with Witch Hazel.

Recipe 4— Hand sanitizer spray with Alcohol and Aloe Vera as primary ingredients

Primary ingredients: Witch Hazel and Aloe Vera
Tools & Equipment

- Small mixing bowl

- Spoon

- Funnel

- Spray bottle (2 ounces)

Ingredients

- 2 ounces of 95% grain Alcohol

- 1 ounce of Aloe Vera

- 1 tsp of Vitamin E oil

- a combination of essential oil (optional)

- Distilled water (or boiled, cooled and filtered)

Combination of essential oils:

- 25 drops of tea tree oil

- 10 drops of lavender essential oil

- 6 drops of lemongrass essential oil

Instructions

1.   Drop all the essential oils plus Vitamin E oil into a small bowl and mix by swirling

2.   Pour Alcohol into the essential oils mix and swirl further

3.   Add Aloe Vera into the mix and whisk the ingredients to achieve a uniform texture.

4.   Put the mixture into the spray bottle and tighten the top

5.   Set for about 30 minutes and then use it when needed.

Advisory notes
Use a colored bottle to avoid intense light interfering with the essential oils in the hand sanitizer. Properly label the container to prevent accidental misuse.

Recipes with Witch Hazel as the main critical ingredient

If you have very dry skin and not extremely vulnerable to risks of infection, then you can use Witch Hazel as a to alcohol.

Recipe 5 – Gel-based hand sanitizer with Witch Hazel and Aloe Vera as primary ingredients

Primary ingredients: Witch Hazel and Aloe Vera

Tools & Equipment

- Small bowl

- Spoon

- Funnel

- Squirt bottle

Ingredients

- 1 ounce of Witch Hazel

- 5 ounce of Aloe Vera gel

- ¼ teaspoon of Vitamin E Oil

- a combination of essential oil (optional)

Combination of essential oils:

- 30 drops of tea tree oil

- 8 drops of lavender essential oil

Instructions

1. Drop all the essential oils into a small bowl and mix by swirling

2.   Pour Witch Hazel into the essential oils mix and swirl further

3.   Add Aloe Vera into the mix and whisk the ingredients to achieve a uniform texture.

4.   Put the mixture into the squirt bottle and tighten the top

5.   Set for about 30 minutes and then use it when needed.

Advisory notes
Use a colored bottle to avoid intense light interfering with the essential oils in the hand sanitizer.

Recipe 6 – Hand sanitizer with Witch Hazel and Aloe Vera as primary ingredients

Primary ingredients: Witch Hazel and Aloe Vera

Tools & Equipment

- Small mixing bowl

- Spoop

- Scooping spoon

- Squeeze bottle

Ingredients

- 1 teaspoon of Witch Hazel

- 8 ounces of Aloe Vera gel

- a combination of essential oil (optional)

Combination of essential oils:

- ¼ teaspoon of Vitamin E Oil

- 30 drops of tea tree oil

- 5 drops lavender essential oil or peppermint

Instructions

1. Mix Witch Hazel, with Aloe Vera oil and Tea tree oil and stir. If the mix is too thin, add some Aloe Vera gel, little by little, to attain the right thickness.
2. Add in essential oils and mix thoroughly

3. Scoop the mixture into the squeeze bottle. Tighten the top after you are finished with pouring.
4. Set for about 30 minutes and then use it when needed.

Advisory notes
Use a colored bottle to avoid strong light interfering with the essential oils in the hand sanitizer.

Recipe 7 – Hand sanitizer spray with Witch Hazel and Aloe Vera as primary ingredients

Primary ingredients: Witch Hazel and Aloe Vera

Tools & Equipment

- Small mixing bowl

- Spoon

- Funnel

- Spray bottle (2 ounces)

Ingredients

- 1 teaspoon of Witch Hazel

- 1 teaspoon of Aloe Vera

- 5 drops of Vitamin E oil

- a combination of essential oil (optional)

- Distilled water (or boiled, cooled and filtered)

Combination of essential oils:

- 5 drops of tea tree oil

- 5 drops of orange essential oil

- 5 drops of lemon essential oil

Instructions

1. Pour all the ingredients except water into the spray bottle. Close the lid and shake gently for about 20 seconds for the mixture to combine.

2. Open the bottle and fill the remaining space with water, leaving some room for shaking. Close the bottle and gently shake for about 15 seconds.

3. Set for about 30 minutes and then use it when needed.

Advisory notes
Use a colored bottle to avoid strong light interfering with the essential oils in the hand sanitizer. Properly label the bottle to avoid accidental misuse.

Recipe 8– Hand sanitizer spray with Witch Hazel and Aloe Vera as primary ingredients

Primary ingredients: Witch Hazel and Aloe Vera

Tools & Equipment

- Small mixing bowl

- Spoon

- Funnel

- Spray bottle (2 ounces)

Ingredients

- 2 ounces of Witch Hazel

- 1 ounce of Aloe Vera

- 1 tsp of Vitamin E oil

- a combination of essential oil (optional)

- Distilled water (or boiled, cooled and filtered)

Combination of essential oils:

- 25 drops of tea tree oil

- 10 drops of lavender essential oil

- 6 drops of lemongrass essential oil

Instructions

1.   Drop all the essential oils plus Vitamin E oil into a small bowl and mix by swirling

2.   Pour Witch Hazel into the essential oils mix and swirl further

3.   Add Aloe Vera into the mix and whisk the ingredients to achieve a uniform texture.

4.   Put the mixture into the spray bottle and tighten the top

5.   Set for about 30 minutes and then use it when needed.

Advisory notes
Use a colored bottle to avoid strong light interfering with the essential oils in the hand sanitizer. Properly label the bottle to avoid accidental misuse.

Recipe 9 – Squeezable hand sanitizer with Witch Hazel and Aloe Vera as primary ingredients

Primary ingredients: Alcohol and Aloe Vera

Tools & Equipment

- Small bowl

- Spoon

- Squeezable bottle

Ingredients

- 2 tablespoons of Witch Hazel

- 3 tablespoons of Aloe Vera gel

- 1/2 teaspoon of Vitamin E Oil

- a combination of essential oil (optional)

Combination of essential oils:

- 20 drops of tea tree oil

- 10 drops of lavender oil

Instructions

1. Drop all the essential oils plus Vitamin E oil into a small bowl and mix by swirling

2. Pour alcohol into the essential oils mix and swirl further

3. Add Aloe Vera into the mix and whisk the ingredients to achieve a uniform texture.

4. Put the mixture into the squeezable bottle and tighten the top

5. Set for about 30 minutes and then use it when needed.

Advisory notes
Use a colored bottle to avoid strong light interfering with the essential oils in the hand sanitizer.

Recipe 10– Gel-based hand sanitizer with Witch Hazel and Aloe Vera as primary ingredients

Primary ingredients: Witch Hazel and Aloe Vera

Tools & Equipment

- Small bowl

- Spoon

- Squirt bottle

Ingredients

- 1 ounce of Witch Hazel

- 5 ounce of Aloe Vera gel

- ¼ teaspoon of Vitamin E Oil

- a combination of essential oil (optional)

Combination of essential oils:

- 5 drops of tea tree oil

- 3 drops of orange essential oil

- 3 drops of clove essential oil

- 3 drops of cinnamon essential oil

- 2 drops of lavender essential oil

Instructions

1. Drop all the essential oils plus Vitamin E oil into a small bowl and mix by swirling

2. Pour Witch Hazel into the essential oils mix and swirl further

3. Add Aloe Vera into the mix and whisk the ingredients to achieve a uniform texture.

4.   Put the mixture into the squirt bottle and tighten the top

5.   Set for about 30 minutes and then use it when needed.

Advisory notes
Use a colored bottle to avoid strong light interfering with the essential oils in the hand sanitizer.

Combo Recipes

Combo recipes refer to those recipes where two or more primary ingredients are blended – either to supplement or complement each other – to boost the efficacy of the final product or gain some additional properties that are in one primary ingredient but lacks in the other(s).

Recipe 11 – Hand sanitizer with Alcohol, Aloe Vera and Glycerin as primary ingredients

Primary ingredients: Alcohol, Aloe Vera and Glycerin

Tools & Equipment

- Mixing bowl

- Spoons

- Cup

- Funnel

- Whisk

- Spray bottle

Ingredients

- 1 tbsp Isopropyl Alcohol

- 2 oz. Aloe Vera

- 1/2 tsp Glycerin

- A combination of essential oils

- Sterile distilled water (or cold boiled water)

  A combination of essential oils:

- 10 drops tea tree oil

- 10 drops cinnamon essential oil

- 5 drops lavender oil (or your preferred scent oil such as lemon oil, peppermint, and lemongrass)

Instructions

1.   Pour alcohol into the mixing bowl.

2.   Add hydrogen peroxide

3.   Add glycerin and then whisk to stir until adequately mixed with a uniform texture

4.   Add essential oils and whisk to stir

5.   Add water and whisk to stir further

6.   Sanitize your bottle using alcohol and hydrogen peroxide leftovers

7.   Pour in the mixture using the funnel

8.   Set for about 30 minutes and then use it when needed.

Advisory notes
If you don't have sterile distilled water, you can use cold boiled water that is filtered. Label the container to avoid accidental use.

Recipe 12 – Spray-based hand sanitizer with Alcohol and Hydrogen Peroxide as primary ingredients

Primary ingredients: Alcohol and Hydrogen

Peroxide Tools & Equipment

- Mixing bowl

- Spoon

- A couple of bottle dispensers (to your preferred size)

Ingredients

- 4 cups of 99% isopropyl alcohol (or 95% ethanol)

- 3 tablespoons of 3% Hydrogen Peroxide

- 2 tablespoons of glycerin

Instructions

1. Pour alcohol into the mixing bowl

2. Add Hydrogen Peroxide
3. Add Glycerin

4. Gently whisk the ingredients

5. Pour the mixed ingredients into the bottle dispensers

6. Set for about 30 minutes and then use it when needed.

Advisory notes
Label the bottles to avoid accidental use.

Recipe 13 – Hand sanitizer with Alcohol, Hydrogen Peroxide, and Aloe Vera as primary ingredients

Primary ingredients: Alcohol, Hydrogen Peroxide and Aloe

Vera Tools & Equipment

- Container

- Pump bottle

Ingredients

- 8 ounces of Isopropyl Alcohol

- ½ ounce of 3% Hydrogen Peroxide

- 1 teaspoon of Aloe Vera

- Sterile distilled water

Instructions

1. Mix all the ingredients except water into a container

2. Add water to bring the total mixture to 11 1/3 cups

3. Set for about 30 minutes and then use it as and when needed.

Advisory notes
If you don't have sterile distilled water, you can use cold boiled water that is filtered. Label the container to avoid accidental use.

Recipe 14 – Spray-based hand sanitizer with Alcohol and Hydrogen Peroxide as primary ingredients

Primary ingredients: Alcohol and Hydrogen Peroxide

Tools & Equipment

- Mixing bowl

- Spoon

- 16 oz. Spray bottle (made of glass)

Ingredients

- 3 ounces of 99% isopropyl alcohol (or 95% ethanol)

- 2 ounces of 5% white vinegar

- 4 ounces of distilled water

- A combination of essential oils

A combination of essential oils:

- 35 drops tea tree oil

- 35 drops cinnamon essential oil

- 10 drops lavender oil (or your preferred scent oil such as lemon oil, peppermint, and lemongrass)

Instructions

1. Drop all the essential oils into a small bowl and mix by swirling

2. Pour alcohol into the essential oils mix and swirl further

3. Add White Vinegar into the mix and whisk the ingredients to achieve a uniform texture.

4. Pour the mixture into the spray bottle and fill up with water

5. Tighten the bottle top and set for about 30 minutes.

6. Use when needed.

Advisory notes
Label the bottles to avoid accidental use.

Mild and Miscellaneous recipes

Mild recipes are those recipes that you can ordinarily use on a daily basis, in the absence of an epidemic. Note, you should not use them when there is an infectious epidemic such as the Corona Virus epidemic or SARS, or MERS or such other derivatives.

Recipe 15 – 'The Secret of Thieves' hand sanitizer

Primary ingredients: Aloe Vera and a combination of essential oils

Tools & Equipment

- Small mixing bowl

- Spoon

- Squeeze bottle (2 ounces)

Ingredients

- 1 tsp of Aloe Vera gel

- 6 ounces of distilled water (or boiled, cooled and filtered)

- a combination of essential oil (optional)

Combination of essential oils:

- 2 drops of Eucalyptus essential oil

- 2 drops of Cinnamon essential oil

- 2 drops of Rosemary essential oil

- 2 drops of Clove essential oil

- 5 drops of lemon oil (or other scent oils such as lavender, peppermint, etc.)

Instructions

1.   Drop all the essential oils into a small bowl and mix by swirling

2.   Add Aloe Vera into the mix and whisk the ingredients to achieve a uniform texture.

3.   Put the mixture into the squeeze bottle and tighten

4.   Set for about 30 minutes and then use it when needed.

Advisory notes
Use a colored bottle to avoid strong light interfering with the essential oils in the hand sanitizer. Properly label the bottle to avoid accidental misuse.

Recipe 16 – Castile Hand Sanitizer

Primary ingredients: Castile soap and Tea tree essential oil

Tools & Equipment

- Small mixing bowl

- Spoon

- Funnel

- Spray bottle

Ingredients

- 1 tsp of Castile soap

- 10 drops of tea tree oil

- 6 ounces of distilled water (or boiled, cooled and filtered)

- ¼ tsp of Vitamin E oil

Instructions

1.   Drop tea tree oil plus Vitamin E oil into a small bowl and mix by swirling

2.   Add castile soap and swirl further

3.   Add water into the mix and stir to achieve a uniform texture.

4.   Put the mixture into the spray bottle and tighten the top

5.   Set for about 30 minutes and then use it when needed.

Advisory notes
Vitamin E oil is used to minimize likely irritation from tea tree oil on sensitive skin. Use a colored bottle to avoid strong light interfering with the essential oils in the hand sanitizer. Properly label the spray bottle to avoid accidental misuse.

Recipe 17 – 'Essentials' hand sanitizer

Primary ingredients: A combination of essential oils Tools & Equipment

- Small mixing bowl

- Spoon

- Spray bottle (2 ounces)

Ingredients

- 2 tsp of Witch Hazel

- distilled water (or boiled, cooled and filtered)

- a combination of essential oil (optional)

Combination of essential oils:

- 6 drops of Eucalyptus essential oil

- 6 drops of Tea tree essential oil

- 6 drops of Lemon oil (or other scent oils such as lavender, peppermint, etc.)

Instructions

1.   Drop all the essential oils into a small bowl and mix by swirling

2.   Put the mixture into the spray bottle

3.   Fill up the spray bottle with distilled water and tighten

4.   Set for about 30 minutes and then use it when needed.

Advisory notes
Use a colored bottle to avoid strong light interfering with the essential oils in the hand sanitizer. Properly label the bottle to avoid accidental misuse.

WHO & CDC Recommended formulation

There are WHO & CDC recommended recipes against Corona Virus (COVID-19). For these various recipes, the ratios and methods are largely the same. Only the quantities vary as per specific needs. There are also slight variations in the quantity of alcohol, based on whether you are using Isopropyl or Ethanol.

Recipe 18 – Hand sanitizer with Alcohol, Hydrogen Peroxide, and Glycerin as primary ingredients

Primary ingredients: Alcohol, Hydrogen Peroxide and Glycerin

Tools & Equipment

- Mixing bowl

- Spoons

- Cup

- Funnel

- Whisk

- Spray bottle

Ingredients

- 8 ounces of Isopropyl Alcohol

- 1 tablespoon of 3% Hydrogen Peroxide

- 1 teaspoon of Glycerin

- Sterile distilled water (or cold boiled water)

Instructions

1. Pour alcohol into the mixing bowl.

2.   Add hydrogen peroxide

3.   Add glycerin and then whisk to stir until properly mixed with a uniform texture

4.   Add water and stir further

5.   Sanitize your bottle using alcohol and hydrogen peroxide leftovers

6.   Pour in the mixture

7.   Set for about 30 minutes and then use it when needed.

Advisory notes
If you don't have sterile distilled water, you can use cold boiled water that is filtered. Label the container to avoid accidental use.

Recipe 19 – Hand sanitizer with Isopropyl Alcohol, Hydrogen Peroxide, and Glycerin as primary ingredients

Primary ingredients: Isopropyl Alcohol, Hydrogen Peroxide, and Glycerin
Tools & Equipment

- Glass/Plastic bottle

- Paddles for mixing (wooden or plastic)

- Measuring jug/cylinder

- Cup

- Funnel

- Whisk

- Alcoholmeter

Ingredients

- 2 gal. of 99% Isopropyl Alcohol
-

- 1.76 cups of 3% Hydrogen Peroxide

- 0.6 cups of 98% Glycerol

- Sterile distilled water (or cold boiled water)

Instructions

1. Pour Isopropyl alcohol into the mixing container.

2. Add hydrogen peroxide

3. Add glycerin and then whisk to stir until properly mixed with a uniform texture

4. Add water and stir further

5. Sanitize your bottle using alcohol and hydrogen peroxide leftovers

6. Pour in the mixture

7. Set for 72 hours and then use it when needed.

Advisory notes
If you don't have sterile distilled water, you can use cold boiled water that is filtered. Label the container to avoid accidental use.

Recipe 20 – Hand sanitizer with Ethanol, Hydrogen Peroxide, and Glycerin as primary ingredients

Primary ingredients: Ethanol, Hydrogen Peroxide and Glycerin Tools & Equipment

- Glass/Plastic bottle

- Paddles for mixing (wooden or plastic)

- Measuring jug/cylinder

- Cup

- Funnel

- Whisk

- Alcoholmeter

Ingredients

- 8333ml of 96% Ethanol

- 417ml of 3% Hydrogen Peroxide

- 145ml of 98% Glycerol

- Sterile distilled water (or cold boiled water)

Instructions

1. Pour Ethanol into the mixing container.

2. Add hydrogen peroxide.

3. Add glycerin and then whisk to stir until properly mixed with a uniform texture.

4. Add water and stir further

5. Sanitize your bottle using alcohol and hydrogen peroxide leftovers

6. Pour in the mixture

7. Set for 72 hours and then use it when needed.

Advisory notes
If you don't have sterile distilled water, you can use cold boiled water that is filtered. Label the container to avoid accidental use.

Recipe 21 – Hand sanitizer with Isopropyl Alcohol, Hydrogen Peroxide, and Glycerin as primary ingredients

Primary ingredients: Isopropyl Alcohol, Hydrogen Peroxide, and Glycerin

Tools & Equipment

- Mixing container (about 2 liters)

- Graduated Glass/Plastic bottle (1000ml)

- Paddles for mixing (wooden or plastic)

- Measuring jug/cylinder

- Cup

- Funnel

- Whisk

- Alcoholmeter

Ingredients

- 751.5ml of 99% Isopropyl Alcohol

- 41.7ml of 3% Hydrogen Peroxide

- 14.5ml of 98% Glycerol

- Sterile distilled water (or cold boiled water)

Instructions

1. Pour Isopropyl alcohol into the mixing container.

2. Add hydrogen peroxide

3. Add glycerin and then whisk to stir until properly mixed with a uniform texture

4. Sanitize your bottle using alcohol and hydrogen peroxide leftovers

5. Pour in the mixture

6.   Add water and stir further

7.   Set for 72 hours and then use it when needed.

Advisory notes
If you don't have sterile distilled water, you can use cold boiled water that is filtered. Label the container to avoid accidental use.

Recipe 22 – Hand sanitizer with Ethanol, Hydrogen Peroxide, and Glycerin as primary ingredients

Primary ingredients: Ethanol, Hydrogen Peroxide and Glycerin Tools & Equipment

- Mixing container (about 2 liters)

- Graduated Glass/Plastic bottle (1000ml)

- Paddles for mixing (wooden or plastic)

- Measuring jug/cylinder

- Cup

- Funnel

- Whisk

- Alcoholmeter

Ingredients

- 833ml of 96% Ethanol

- 41.7ml of 3% Hydrogen Peroxide

- 14.5ml of 98% Glycerol

- Sterile distilled water (or cold boiled water)

Instructions

1.   Pour Ethanol into the mixing container.

2.   Add hydrogen peroxide

3.   Add glycerin and then whisk to stir until properly mixed with a uniform texture

4.   Sanitize your bottle using alcohol and hydrogen peroxide leftovers

5.   Pour in the mixture

6.   Add water and stir further

7.   Set for 72 hours and then use it when needed.

Advisory notes
If you don't have sterile distilled water, you can use cold boiled water that is filtered. Label the container to avoid accidental use.

PART III: TIPS & FAQS

Just to add a cap to your knowledge and skills… and in addition to your recipes, I have prepared you a dessert of tips and facts to consolidate your competence.

Seize them up. Keep them at your fingertips.

Tips

To help you have an easy time preparing, using, and safeguarding your hand sanitizer, I have come up with the following important tips that you ought to put on your fingertips.

Tips for dealing with acute infections such as COVID-19 COVID-19 or other such coronavirus infections require extra-ordinary sanitary care. Thus, you have to take extra-ordinary measures that you wouldn't necessarily need to take under normal circumstances.

The following are tips specifically tailored to deal with COVID-19 and similar infections.

Do:

1.   Wash your hands thoroughly and frequently

2.   Ensure that your home-made hand sanitizer contains at least 60% alcohol

3.   Ensure that your hands are completely dry before applying hand sanitizer

4.   Quarantine your home-made hand sanitizer for 72 hours before use – this allows hydrogen peroxide to penetrate the spores and kill them.

Don't:

1.   Apply hand sanitizer on wet hands

2.   Apply hand sanitizer on oily hands

3.   Rely on hand sanitizers that have only essential oils

4.   Put your faith in antibacterial wipes

5.   Put your faith in baby wipes as an alternative to hand sanitizers

6.   Take hand sanitizer as an alternative to washing hands with soap in running water. Hand sanitizer should be considered in cases where there is no soap and clean running water.

Tips on essential oils

We've already seen the benefits of essential oils. We've also seen how to use them in various recipes.

The following are general tips to keep in mind in as far as essential oils for hand sanitizer are concerned:

1.   To boost antiseptic efficacy, add cinnamon, peppermint, clove, and lavender essential oils to your recipe. These oils have antiseptic properties.
2.   To have an appealing scent, add any of the essential oils with fragrance properties. These include lavender, peppermint, and rosemary, among others.

Tips on making your hand sanitizer soft on your skin

We've already seen how critical it is to keep your hands free from dryness. Dryness promotes skin cracking. These cracks become easy avenues for fresh infections. Making your hand sanitizer soft on your skin will not only kill existing germs but also help prevent new germs from penetrating.

To achieve this:

1.   Add Vitamin E oil to your ingredients. Vitamin E Oil has an ameliorating effect on your skin. This helps to mitigate the harsh effect of alcohol or hydrogen peroxide

2.   Use Aloe Vera or Glycerin as one of your base ingredients

Tips on avoiding irritation and allergies

Each skin has its unique sensitivity depending on genetic, metabolic, and environmental factors. Due to this sensitivity, some people are likely to be more susceptible to irritation and allergies concerning certain ingredients than others.

To mitigate such irritations and allergies:

1.   If you feel irritated by alcohol, substitute it with Witch Hazel. You can also add Aloe Vera.

2.   If you are allergic to Aloe Vera, substitute it with Glycerin

3.   If you are allergic to most of the essential oils, substitute them with either olive oil or grapeseed oil

Tips on disinfecting your hand sanitizer utensils

When making your hand sanitizer, it is important to ensure that the utensils that you are using are disinfected.

To achieve this:

1. Pour some 3% hydrogen peroxide and spread evenly along the surface that is going to interact with your ingredients. You may need to swirl or spray, whichever the case.

2.   You can also use kitchen bleach instead of hydrogen peroxide

Tips on what to do if you lack some essential ingredients

Depending on your locality, some ingredients may not be easily available. On the other hand, during a pandemic such as COVID-19, some ingredients may get depleted from the shop shelves.

To ensure that you are not hampered by lack of certain ingredients in your endeavor to make the hand sanitizer, consider the following tips:

1.   In case you don't have 99% Isopropyl alcohol or 95% ethanol, then use alcohol that is at least 60% proof as hand sanitizer. Don't mix it with anything. After sanitizing your hand, you can use normal lotion to prevent dryness.

2.   Use alternative substitutes. For example, if there is no alcohol, use Witch hazel; if there is no Aloe Vera, use glycerin; if both alcohol and Witch hazel are not there, use 3% hydrogen peroxide or 5% white vinegar.

Tips on safety and quality control

Safety and quality control are important in ensuring the efficacy of your hand sanitizer. This is extremely important during a pandemic situation, such as that occasioned by SARS.

Poor quality ingredients or lack of safety considerations can harm more than it benefits.

To ensure safety and quality controls:

1.   Use Alcoholmeter to verify the volume of alcohol

2.   Eliminate potential contaminating spores using hydrogen peroxide

3.   Use humectants such as glycerol to improve the acceptability of other ingredients.

4.   Keep your hand sanitizer out of reach of small children – they may decide to ingest it.

5.   Label your hand sanitizer to avoid accidental use

6.   Use a dark-colored bottle in case the ingredients include essential oils. Essential oils are susceptible to strong light and thus can lose their efficacy.
7.   To disinfect hand sanitizer bottles before pouring the sanitizer, soak them in 1000 ppm chlorine for at least 15 minutes and then thoroughly rinse with distilled water before use. Let the bottles dry completely before pouring in the sanitizer.
8.   For protection against coronavirus, use WHO/CDC recommended ingredients and proportions. Don't add ingredients that have not been recommended, such as essential oils and vitamin E oil, as they may negatively affect the efficacy of the sanitizer.

9.   Make sure your source your ingredients are from a reputable supplier.

Tips on how to use your hand sanitizer
Hand sanitizer is easy to use. Thus, there is nothing extra-ordinary about its usage. However, there are certain simple things, if overlooked, can result in suboptimal use.

To ensure optimal use:

1.   Understand that hand sanitizer is no substitute for washing your hands with soap and clean running water.

2.   Rub the hand sanitizer for about 20 seconds or until your hands are dry (you may wipe off excess sanitizer with a dry cloth, but make sure that the cloth is sanitized)

3.   In case of an epidemic, put your hand sanitizer in a portable bottle so that you can carry it and use it in places where there is no running water and soap.

FAQs

1. Can I use vodka as an alternative to Isopropyl alcohol?

Yes and No. Most vodka is just about 70% proof or even less. And even if it is higher, it doesn't have the kind of alcohol found in Isopropyl or ethanol. Under normal circumstances, you can use vodka. But, when there is an epidemic such as COVID-19, vodka won't be as effective since CDC and WHO recommends alcohol with a content of at least 91% to blend with other ingredients such as Glycerin (and even Aloe Vera) and Hydrogen Peroxide, yet retain at least 60% alcohol content in the final mixture. The 70% Vodka won't suffice.

2. Is Witch Hazel as effective as alcohol?

Though Witch Hazel is an alternative to alcohol, it is less than par. It should only be an alternative when alcohol is not available or for cases where there is no serious pandemic such as COVID-19.

3.   Can I make a hand sanitizer without Aloe Vera and essential oils?

Yes. You can use Aloe Vera alternatives such as glycerin. Even without Aloe Vera alternatives, you can simply use water as the base ingredient. Essential oils are optional. As you may have realized, WHO & CDC haven't recommended essential oils in their formulation – that is, in the case of COVID-19.

4.   How long can the hand sanitizer last without getting spoilt?

Alcohol works as a preservative. As such, due to the effect of alcohol, hand sanitizer can last for a couple of months without getting spoilt.

5. How can I mute the smell of alcohol?

Unless you are making the WHO/CDC recommended formulation, you can use essential oils that have a strong fragrance to mute the smell of alcohol. Such essential oils include lavender and peppermint, among others.

6. I am allergic to Aloe Vera, what should I do?

If you are allergic to Aloe Vera, you can use its alternatives, such as glycerin.

7.   How can I stop my hands from feeling dry and irritated due to the effect of alcohol?

To ensure that alcohol does not adversely dry your skin, add Aloe Vera and Vitamin E Oil. If you cannot use Aloe Vera, then use Glycerin.

8. Where can I get the ingredients?

Most of the ingredients are easily available over the counter – either at pharmacies or beauty/cosmetic shops.

9. Can't I just wipe my hands with plain alcohol or its alternatives?

Yes, you can – for so long as you meet the recommended concentration levels. However, plain alcohol or hydrogen can cause excessive dryness, thus leading to irritation. This can also cause further infection as the skin becomes cracked. Thus, to avoid this excessive dryness, itching, and irritability, use of Aloe Vera, glycerin, Vitamin E oil, and some essential oils are advised.

10.   Does mixing Aloe Vera with Witch Hazel in the same solution hurt?

No. It only makes the solution stronger and more effective. However, unless under a serious epidemic such as COVID-19, it may simply be overkill for ordinary use.

FACE MASK

A face mask filters the particles carried by air, and it can help to reduce our exposure to air pollution, germs, and so on. A high-quality facial mask filters particles as small as PM2.5, but they do not protect against the gases, often toxic, that pollute our cities, such as those emitted by diesel vehicles.

In the market you can find a massive range of Face Masks, are you confused?

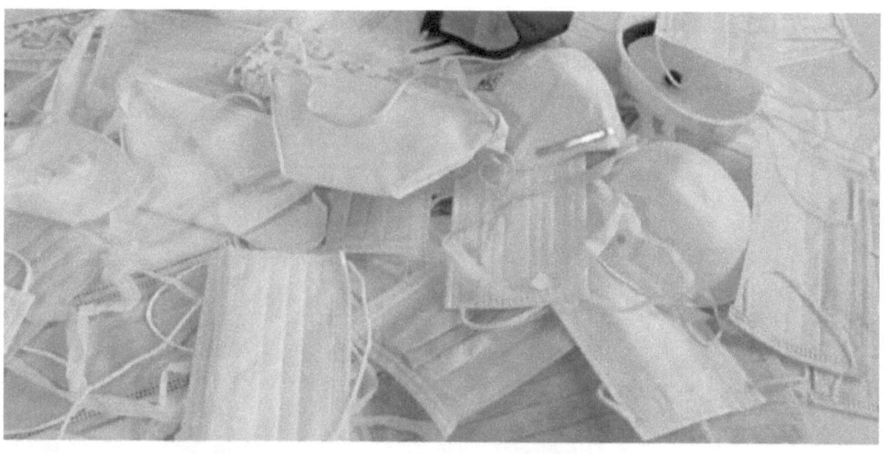

You can find help on some websites on how to decide which is the best mask for you and your family, and you can find a lot of reviews that will give you a good idea of what to look for when buying a mask. Here is a summary of these features:

a) Presence of a multilayer filter, able to filter better

b) Eu or US Certified Mask

c)	Correctly fitting of the model fits on our face, it is critical (Nouse, left and right sides

The certification indicates the mask has been tested and meets the reference standards for filtering small dispersed aero particles. In the market, you can find a mask with EU and or the US certification and classification

MASK CLASSIFICATION

The EU classification

The FFP2 or FFP3 classification, for example, is an assessment standard tested by the European Union. Therefore, orient yourself on masks compliant with the relevant standard, EN149. Which defines 3 classes of filtering efficiency for this type of mask: FFP1, FFP2, FFP3

a.   FFP1 masks: they are commonly considered "dust-proof" masks, have a filtering efficiency of 78% and are insufficient to protect against coronavirus;

b.   FFP2 and FFP3 masks: they have a filtering efficiency of 92% and 98% respectively and are both recommended for those who must defend themselves from the virus such as doctors, nurses and health personnel ;

The US classification

Classification N95, N99, or N100 is a certification approved by the United States government at the National Institute for Safety and Health at Work (NIOSH) of the United States Centers for Disease Control and Prevention (CDC). The NIOSH N95 certification, for example, means that the mask should filter 95% of the particles above 0.3 microns, which is a much smaller size than PM 2.5. N99 respirators filter more or less 99% of these particles.

N100 masks are difficult to find; you may contact an industrial supplier to get them. The difference between the P100 and N100 masks (or, more generally, between the "P" and the "N") is that the P can also filter the pollutants deriving from oil.

Efficacy one must wear them correctly

To have a minimum of effectiveness, the mouth and nose must be completely isolated from the outside. It is, therefore, vital that you choose a mask of the correct size, as each one will position itself on the face in a slightly different way.

Make sure the mask fits well

It is critical to make sure t hat the mask fits tightly and that there are no empty spaces to let in the outside air. Any gap at the edges of the mask would allow the air to completely neutralize any benefit or protection that would be obtained from filtering the polluting particles, no matter how expensive or trendy or of a good brand. This is, therefore, a minimum condition - necessary but not sufficient - to have some protection.

The eye-glasses test

A good test for eyeglass wearers is if the glasses mist up due to the steam when wearing the mask. If so, the masks are not airtight, which passes from the edges between the mask and the skin of the face.

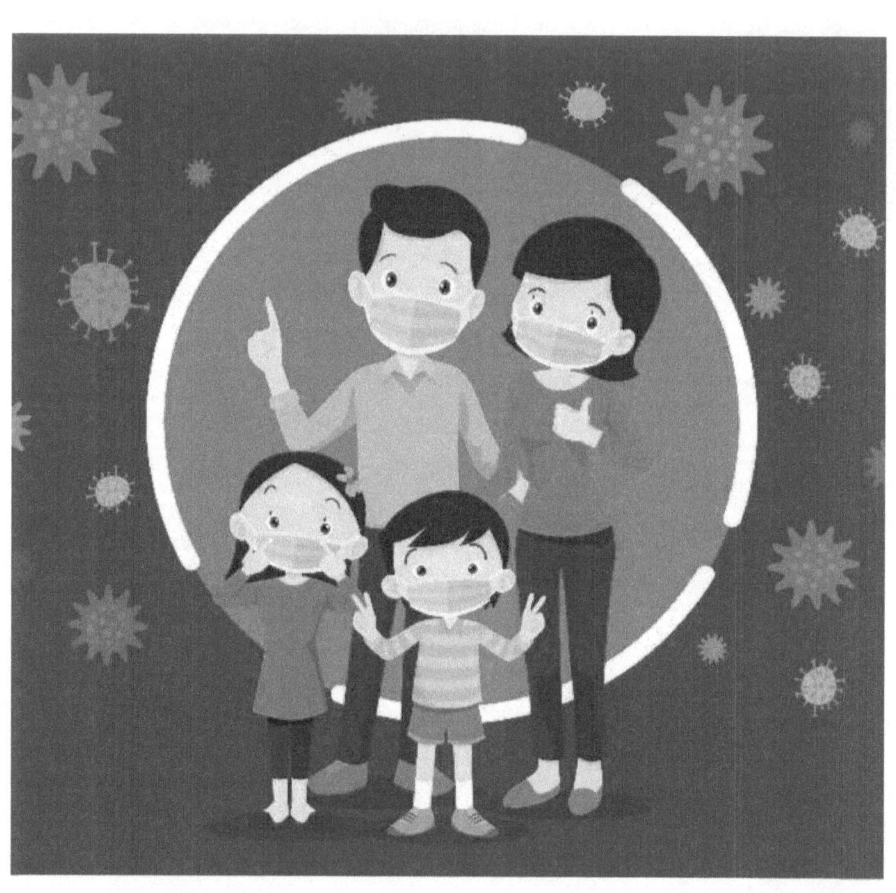

Respiratory Protection

A protective mask may reduce the spread of infection, but it will not eliminate the risk, particularly when a disease has more than 1 route of transmission. A mask, no matter how efficient at filtration or how good the seal, will have minimal effect if it is not used in conjunction with other preventative measures, such as:

-    isolation of infected cases,

-    immunization,

-    good respiratory etiquette,

-    regular hand hygiene.

The filter masks protect against inhalable dust, fumes and mists of liquids (aerosols), but not from steam and gas. The protective mask, filtering Face Mask, should cover the nose and mouth, and it is built with different filter materials and the mask itself. These masks are generally prescribed in the workplace where the exposure air limit value is exceeded.

Remember to follow the supplier cautions and limitations: for instance do not use if the atmosphere has less then 19,5% of oxygen, and do not use in a dangerous atmosphere.

The different types of masks.

- Masks to create a physical barrier protecting the others from ourselves

- Masks to protect ourselves from external factors, individual protection.

Masks to protect others from ourselves –(Type Surgical Mask)

Typically they are those of gauze used by healthcare professionals and surgeons to prevent saliva droplets from falling on the operative field. The Medical / surgical are regulated under USA ASTM F2100 21 CFR 878.4040.

They are used to prevent the sick from spreading the infection, but they do not protect the healthy from the disease. Also useful to doctors and healthcare professionals to avoid droplets of saliva from falling on patients; They serve to protect patients. So they don't help to protect the healthy who is wearing them. They have no protection against the virus that penetrates through those sheets of gauze and therefore do not protect.

Masks to Protect ourselves Respiratory Mask (Individual protection devices/equipment)

These are high-quality respiratory protection devices suitable for the professional environment. They primarily serve to protect against fine particles, dust, and various viruses, fumes and mists of inhalable liquids (aerosols), but not from steam and gas. Their effectiveness is assessed based on the filtration rate but also based on the internal leakage rate.

The Ffp2 and Ffp3 masks are those equipped with a filter. These truly protect but must only be used by healthcare professionals who treat infectious patients and by law enforcement officers who, in certain circumstances, may be in contact with the sick.

Masks Requirements by Type and Level

BFE= Bacteria Filtration Efficiency

PFE= Particle Filtration Efficiency

0,3 Micron: the most challenging size particle to be captured

SURGICAL MASK			Level 1	Level 2	Level 3
Surgical Mask	USA ASTM F2100	BFE	>95%	>98%	>98%
		PFE	>95%	>98%	>98%
	EU : EN 14683	PFE	>95%	>98%	>98%

RESPIRATORY MASK			Level 1	Level 2	Level 3
	Usa : NIOSH(42 CR 84)		N95	N99	N100
		0,3 Micron	>95%	>99%	>99,7%
			FFP1	FFP2	FFP3
	EU: EN 149: 2001	0,3 Micron	>80%	>94%	>95%

EU has been working on updating the standard to align with the US since 2013

How to Choose my Respiratory Mask?

Each type of disposable protection mask has different characteristics it is possible to summarize in this table:

Protection level	1	2	3
Contaminant	**Fine particles and powders** (silica, glass wool, graphite, cement, sulfur, coal, ferrous metal shavings, wood, etc.).	**Fine and toxic particles** (quartz, metal shavings, molds, bacteria, etc.).	**Dangerous and carcinogenic particles** (asbestos, viruses, spores, pesticides, lead, cement, etc.).
use	Perfect for DIY and work in various sectors: textile industry, crafts, metallurgy, carpentry, etc.	Ideal for a variety of jobs in different industries: wastewater treatment, waste disposal, mines, quarries, metalworking.	Ideal for those who work in contact with **asbestos** (in a concentration of less than 1 fiber / cm3 in 1 hour) or **legionella** (short-term intervention). Protects against pollen and **viruses**.
Presence or absence of the valve	Available with or without valve	Available with or without valve	Always equipped with a valve

Essential characteristics are the valve on a mask has numerous advantages:

1. greater comfort,
2. absence of condensation inside the mask,
3. no fogging of the glasses,
4. prevents respiratory resistance, helping to breathe in and out quickly.

If your doctor tells you to put them on because, for example, you are a person potentially at risk or you can infect your family members, then they should be used. Otherwise, the mask is not needed. It is much more useful to wash your hands.

Available masks block them but must be used by healthcare professionals. Those who well do not need to wear a mask. Those who must strictly put on the mask, even the surgical one, are those who are sick.

What is the corona Virus?

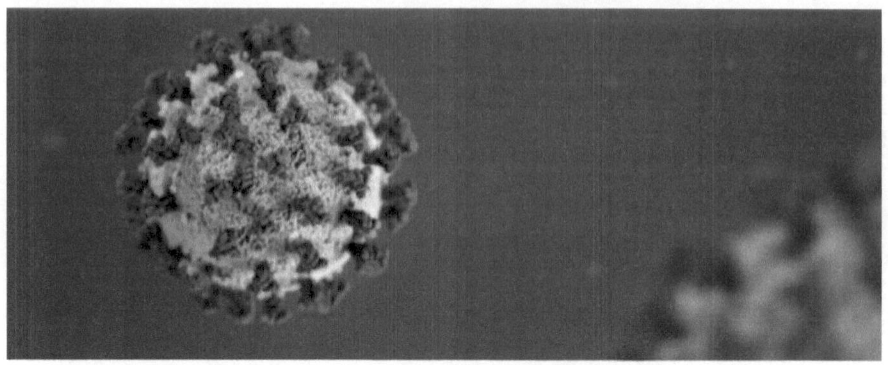

The coronaviruses belong to the "coronaviridae" RNA virus family due to the morphological aspect of the viral particle. In essence, they are round viruses of 120-130 nanometers in diameter, with spicules on the surface that form a sort of a crown.

Coronavirus is a family that contains more than 100 different species of viruses, which infect birds, animals, including mammals and even humans. We knew only 6 that infected humans, 4 are the common cold viruses.

We had zoonotic infections that passed from animal to man since 2002, they are coronaviruses.

-       In 2002 SARS, which is a severe acute respiratory syndrome with a mortality of 10%, i

-       In 2012, the MERS acute "Middle Eastern" syndrome, in Saudi Arabia, with the death of 35%.

-       In December 2019, this new coronavirus.

All these viruses are transmitted from animal to man; this is called Zoonosis: an infection that primarily affects an animal and can also spread to humans despite not being its natural host.

How Small is a Virus and a Coronavirus?

To have an idea about the size of a virus it useful to compare it with another well now small particles we commonly knew, the graphic will give

you a better Idea

- 1/25,4 Inch = 1000 μm (microns)

- Pm 10 = 10 μm (microns) = 1/2540 Inch

- Red Blood cell = 7 μm (microns)

- Bacteria = 0,6 μm (microns)

- Virus = 0,2 μm (microns)

- Coronavirus = 0,150/0,200 μm (microns)

- Bacteriophage MS2 virus = 0.023 μm (microns)

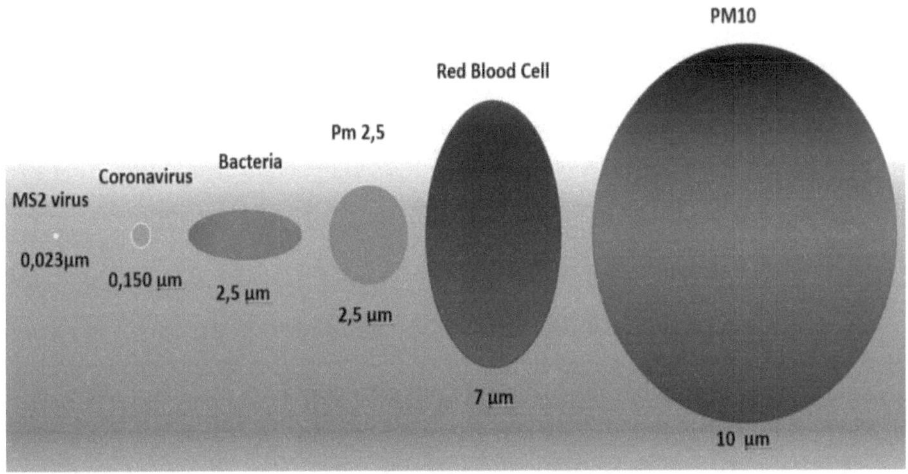

How a Virus can be transmitted:
Studies are underway to better understand how Covid 19 virus is transmitted.

A virus can be transferred from one person to one or more persons, such as close contact with persons infected, i.e., among family members or in a healthcare environment.

The new Coronavirus is a respiratory disease that mainly spreads through close contact with a sick person. The primary route is the droplets of the breath of infected people, for example through:

- Saliva, coughing, and sneezing
- Direct personal contact with the hands, by touching contaminated hands with mouth, nose or eyes.
- In rare cases, the infection can occur through fecal contamination.

The respiratory disease is not transmitted by food, We recommend to respect good hygiene practices handling food. Remember to avoid contact between raw and cooked food.

According to WHO, the main route of transmission of the virus, based on currently available data, is through close contact with symptomatic people, what is close contact?

Close contact can be defined as:

- A person living in the same house like a virus case;

- A person who has had direct physical contact with a virus case (e.g., handshake);

- A person who has had unprotected direct contact with the secretions of a virus case (for example, touching used handkerchiefs with bare hands);

- A person who was in a closed space with a case of virus (e.g., meeting room, classroom, hospital waiting room), at a distance of fewer than 2 meters;

- A person who had direct (face-to-face) contact with a case of a virus, less than 2 meters away and lasting longer than 15 minutes;

-	A healthcare professional or other person providing direct assistance to a case of virus or laboratory staff involved in handling samples of a case of the virus without the use of recommended PPE or through the use of unsuitable PPE;

-	A person who has traveled by plane sitting in the two adjacent seats, in any direction, close to a person affected by a virus
-	travel companions or assistance persons and crewmembers assigned to the section of the plane where the case index was seated.

Can the infection be contracted from a case without symptoms?

Yes! It is possible, although in rare cases, that people in the prodromal stages of the disease, and therefore with absent or very mild symptoms, can transmit the virus.

Who is most at risk of getting the infection?

People who have traveled or live into areas at risk of infection or people who meet the criteria of close contact with a confirmed or probable case of the virus.

Can healthcare professionals be at risk of being infected by new Coronavirus?

Yes, they can be. All healthcare professionals come into contact with many patients, and this more often than the other population does.

World Health Organization (WHO) recommends to all healthcare professionals to apply appropriate control and prevention measures to avoid any infections in general and respiratory diseases in particular.

How can we prevent or mitigate the risk of infection?

To prevent the risk of infection with a virus, it is a priority to take care of hand hygiene and respiratory secretions. The World Health Organization is recommending to wear a mask only if:

-	You suspect having contracted the new coronavirus and experience symptoms such as coughing or sneezing,

-	You are caring of a person alleged to be infected.

One of the suggested measures is to wear a protective mask

Wearing a mask helps to limit the spread of the virus to other people. But has to be adopted in addition to other measures the hand hygiene and surface Hygiene. WHO informs that the mask is not necessary for the general population in the absence of symptoms of respiratory diseases. Basic protective measures against the new coronavirus (https://www.who.int/emergencies/diseases/novel-coronavirus-2019/advice-for-public) . Coronavirus disease (COVID-19) advice for the public: When and how to use masks (https://www.who.int/emergencies/diseases/novel-coronavirus-2019/advice-for-public/when-and-how-to-use-masks)

When to use a mask according to WHO recommendation

-        If you are healthy, you only need to wear a mask if you are taking care of a person with the suspected 2019-nCoV infection.
-        Wear a mask if you are coughing or sneezing.

-        Masks are valid only when used in combination with frequent hand-cleaning with alcohol-based hand rub or soap and water.

-        If you wear a mask, then you must know how to use it and dispose of it properly.

How to put on, use, take off and dispose of a mask:

-        Before putting on a mask, clean hands with alcohol-based hand rub or soap and water.

-        Cover mouth and nose with mask and make sure there are no gaps between your face and the mask.

-        Avoid touching the mask while using it; if you do, clean your hands with alcohol-based hand rub or soap and water.

-        Replace the mask with a new one as soon as it is damp and do not re-use single-use masks.

-        To remove the mask: remove it from behind (do not touch the front of a mask); discard immediately in a closed bin; clean hands with alcohol-based hand rub or soap and water.

How to Wear a Mask WHO directions:

-       Before putting on the mask,

-       First. Wash your hands with soap and hot water or with an alcoholic solution 60%.

-       Second. Cover your nose and mouth with the mask making sure it fits snugly on your face.

-       Remember to avoid touching the mask while you wear it, if you touch it, wash your hands.

-       When a mask gets wet, you must replace it with a new one, do not reuse it if that mask is single-use masks

How to Remove the mask WHO directions

-       Follow the suggested recommendation and directions

-       Taking the mask from the elastic band

-       Do not touch the front of the mask;

-       Throw it immediately in a closed bag

-       Wash your hands.

https://www.who.int/emergencies/diseases/novel-coronavirus-2019/advice-for-public/when-and-how-to-use-masks

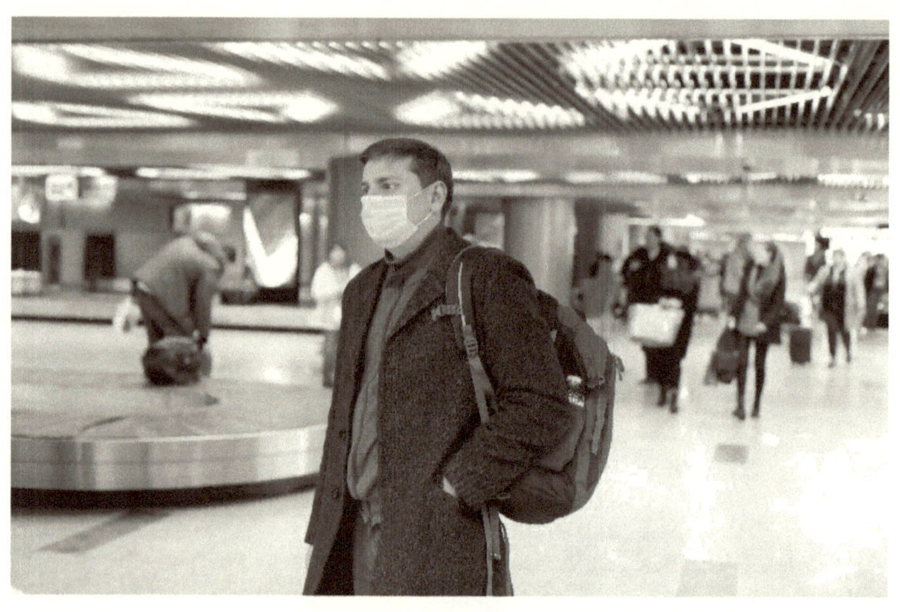

Homemade mask DIY

We would not recommend the use of homemade face masks as a method of reducing transmission of infection from aerosols.

Researchers think that a homemade mask should only be considered as a last resort, the last possible option to reduce droplet transmission, better than no protection.

When masks are sold out, or they cannot be found in the store and are sold on the web with biblical delivery times, do-it-yourself masks are the last a solution. Masks made with simple materials within everyone's reach.

Mask DIY is a turmoil on the web! You can find tutorials of all kinds of material on the internet. One of the models is made with parchment paper. There are also improvised masks made with bras cups. The most refined resort to the cloth masks, made with two rectangles of cotton, one knitted and two pieces of tubular elastic. And some use paper napkins or kitchen rolls. Two tears, a stapling stroke, and two rubber bands, and you're done.

The effectiveness of these masks, however, is all worth trying.

On the web, you find videos of homemade masks with different creative and technical variations, including those made with two pieces of cotton or TNT fabric sewn together by machine after being cut out on a pattern prepared by the same tutorials.

However, experts suggest paying attention to a DIY that, if clumsy, can affect the effectiveness of the mask.

Homemade masks can only act as a last option for those who don't have any equipment but must protect themselves. **They can never be a replacement for surgical/medical masks.**

Remember that gauze masks are used to prevent the surgeon's droplets from falling, but people who are not infected with Coronavirus are useless. "It's just paranoia that healthy people use improperly."

Which are the Best Materials for a Homemade DIY Mask

We want to introduce to you exciting research where the Researchers selected a range of household materials useful for homemade masks and tested the capacity to capture virus-sized particles in comparison to a surgical mask.

Abstract: This study examined homemade masks as an alternative to commercial face masks. Several household materials were evaluated for the capacity to block bacterial and viral aerosols. Twenty-one healthy volunteers made their own face masks from cotton t-shirts; the masks were then tested for fit. The number of microorganisms isolated from coughs of healthy volunteers wearing their homemade mask, a surgical mask, or no mask was compared using several air-sampling techniques. The median-fit factor of the homemade masks was one-half that of the surgical masks. Both masks significantly reduced the number of microorganisms expelled by volunteers, although the surgical mask was 3 times more effective in blocking transmission than the homemade mask. Our findings suggest that a homemade mask should only be considered as a last resort to prevent droplet transmission from infected individuals, but it would be better than no protection. (Disaster Med Public Health Preparedness. 2013; 0: 1-6). (

Davies, Anna & Thompson, Katy-Anne & Giri, Karthika & Kafatos, George & Walker, James & Bennett, Allan. (2013). Testing the Efficacy of Homemade Masks: Would They Protect in a Pandemic Influence ?. Disaster medicine and public health preparedness. 7. 413-418. 10.1017 / dmp.2013.43.)

The test was performed to see how well those different materials coped with selected bacteria and viruses. For this research, the researcher decided 2 pathogens:

- The Bacillus atrophaeus bacteria (0.93-1.25 microns in size),

- The Bacteriophage MS2 virus (0.023 microns in size).

In this research, the selected materials Vs. a surgical mask is the follows:
- Vacuum cleaner Bag

- Tea Towel

- Cotton Mix

- Cotton T-Shirt 100%

- Antimicrobial Pillow

- Scarf

- Pillowcase

- Linen

- Silk

The question is: can homemade masks capture smaller viruses?

To answer this question, we select the test vs. Bacteriophage MS2 particles that 0.02 micron, which is 5 times smaller than the common Virus.

The research results face out all of the homemade materials managed to capture 50% of virus particles or more. The Vacuum cleaner Bag and a Double layer of tea Towels have a filter capacity close to a Surgery Mask**, but BREATH wearing A Vacuum cleaner bag or 2 tea**

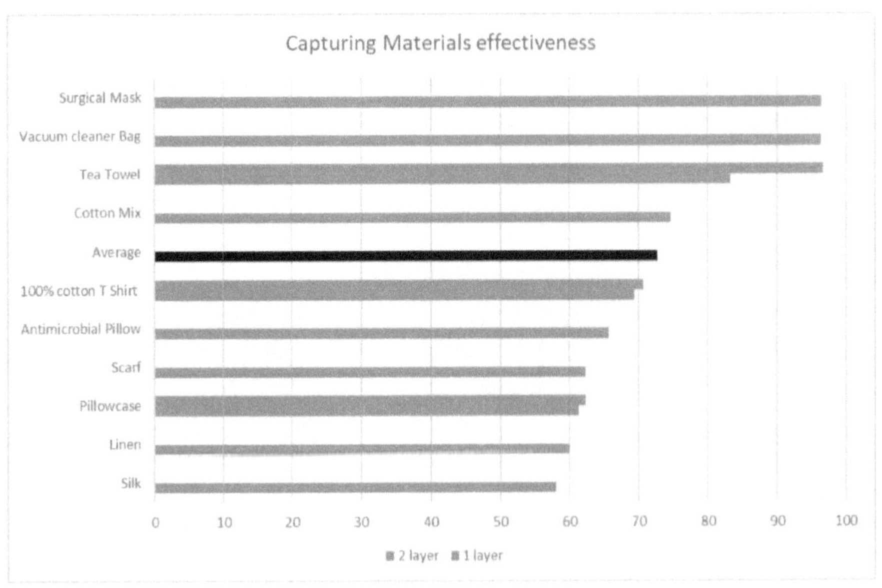

% capturing Material Effectiveness		
Material	1 layer	2 layer
Surgical Mask	96,45	
Vacuum cleaner Bag	96,35	
Tea Towel	83,24	96,71
Cotton Mix	74,60	
Average	72,72	
100% cotton T Shirt	69,42	70,66
Antimicrobial Pillow	65,62	
Scarf	62,30	
Pillowcase	61,28	62,38
Linen	60,00	
Silk	58,00	

My Consideration: Has more Effective Two-Layered Masks?

The scientists tested virus-size particles against the tea towel, pillowcase, and 100% cotton shirt double-layered. As you can see, double layers didn't help so much.

The Vacuum cleaner Bag and a Double layer of tea Towels have a filter capacity close to a Surgery Mask**, how conformable and how easy it breathing wearing A Vacuum cleaner bag or 2 tea towel layers mask: the comfortability depend by the time you will wear them, and the breathability it is not easy!**

DIY Face Mask an Overview

The surgical mask is used to reduce the emission of viremia by those who are infected or healthy carriers, so they are not used to avoid transposing the virus but are used to prevent spreading the virus.

Even a mask can be used to avoid /reduce the virus spreads if it covers the nose and mouth, blocking the drops of saliva, which are carriers of the virus externally to the respiratory tract of the also infected a healthy or unknown infected carrier.

If everyone wore masks, there would be a drastic reduction in viremia.

Homemade masks are only a temporary solution and can act as a last option for those who do not have access to any equipment but must protect themselves.

They can never be a replacement for surgical masks.

Without your mask, remember that this is only a temporary solution and that it absolutely does not replace the surgical one.

The University of Hong Kong Temporary Mask SolutionInsert

Hong Kong-Shenzhen Hospital and the Science Park have recently developed a do-it-yourself method, but have stressed that "they cannot be considered as permanent solutions". To make a mask, the materials are:

- Kitchen Paper

- Resistant tissue paper,

- Rubber bands

- A hole punch

- Tape 2 inch Wide

- Binder clips

- Scissors

\-   Plastic Coated Wires

\-   Moldable iron wire coated in plastic,

The Hong Kong-Shenzhen Hospital has also specified that the materials, including transparent film, filter for air conditioners, and cotton cloths, are not suitable for making masks.

Here are the indications on how to proceed:

A)   Wash your hands thoroughly with soap.

B)   Wash and sterilize the tools you will be working with.

C)   Overlap two kitchen paper napkins

D)   Place a piece of tissue paper, which will act as the bottom layer of the mask, over the two parts of kitchen paper

E)   Cut the napkin in two to create a rectangle

F)   Use the paper tape to seal the two sides of the mask

G)   Drill two holes on each side sealed with the perforator

H)   Attach the metal wire with paper tape on the upper edge of the mask to create a bridge for the nose

I)   Tie four elastic bands through the holes formed on the sides of the mask

Homemade Face Mask an example of DIY

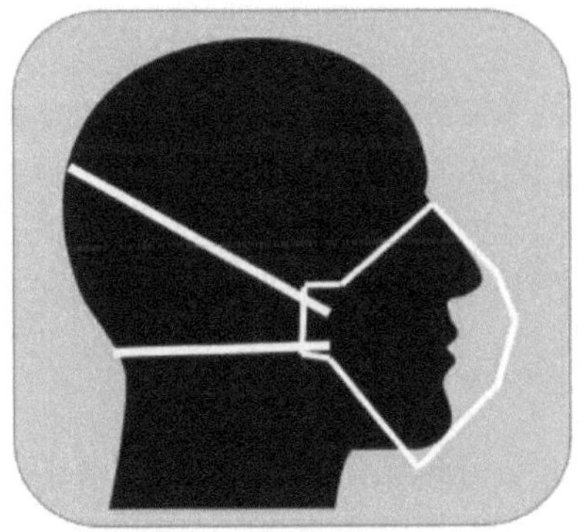

Material

-   Scissor

-   Material (do not use old and used material)

-   Paper Pattern

-   a hole punch (for hard material)

-   Sewing machine or hand Sewing with needle yarn

-   Plastic Coated Wires

-   Adhesive Tape 1 inch wide

A)   1. Nose Moldable iron wire coated in plastic, the metallic wire with

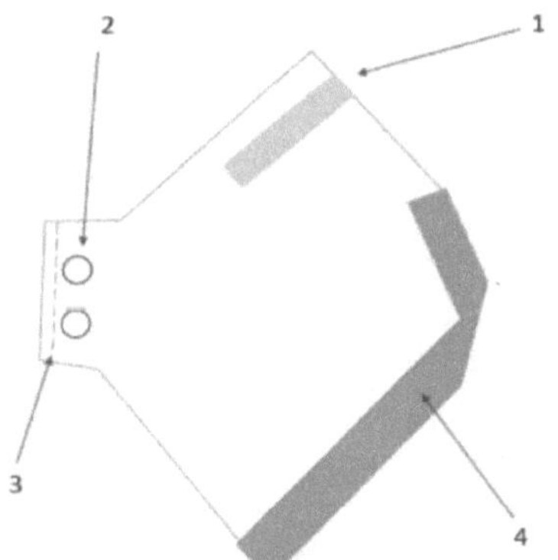
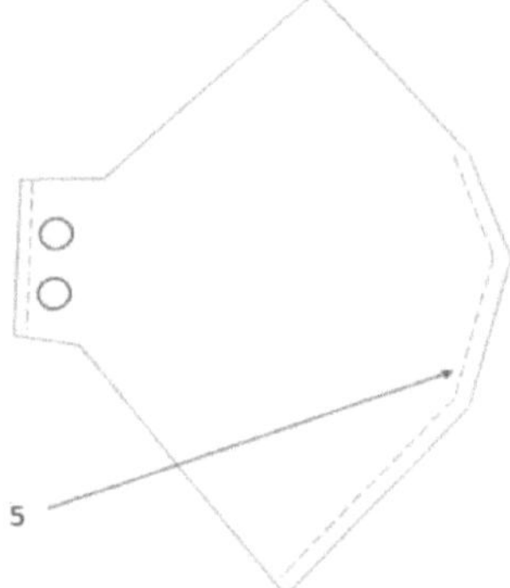

paper tape to make the nose bridge wire

B)   Holes for the band

C)   Double robust sewing

D)   Adhesive Tap Band

E)   Swing to link the 2 sides it under the Adhesive tape

1 create a Paper Pattern

Desing in a wite paper this pattern which will be used to cut out the bag material here is the example with 3 size

Large

Medium

Smal

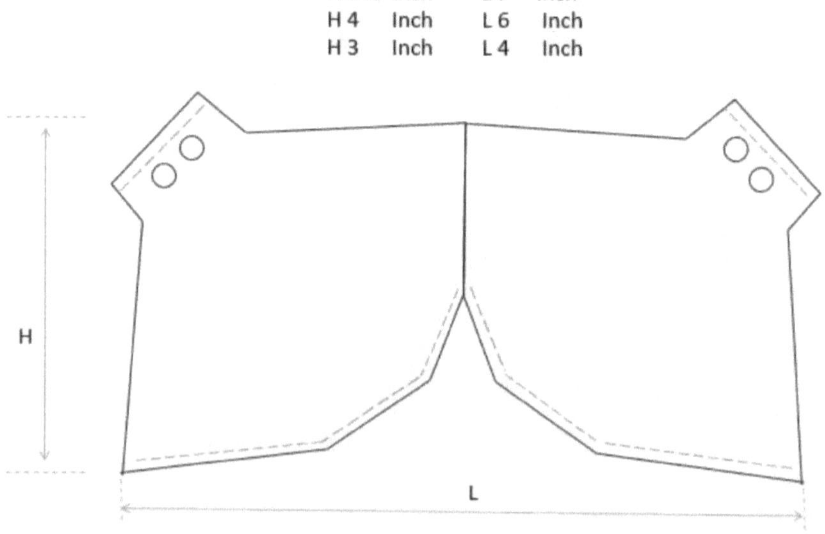

2. Cut prepare the sheared

Cut following the lines. Do not worry if a perfect job will not succeed; the aim is to allow you to take minimal precautions for your health, not bad for aesthetics. You will see that already from the second mask, much more familiarity, therefore, do not lose heart!

1 Cut the filter material following the paper pattern
2 Make the holes
3 Apply the Moldable iron wire coated in plastic,for the nouse use the tape

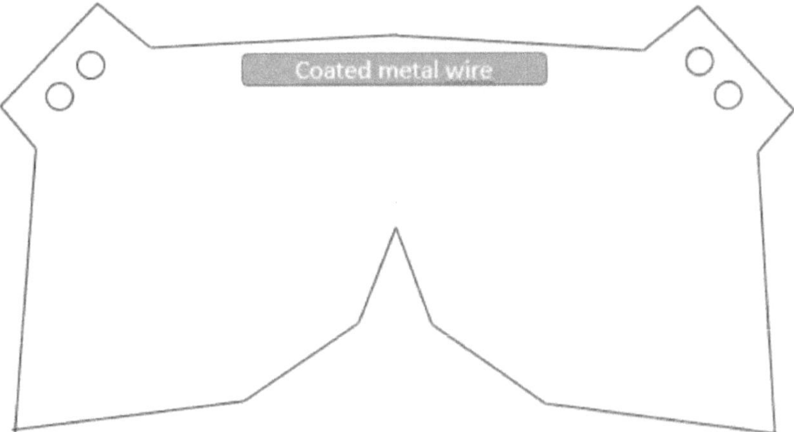

3. Assembling

Then move on to sewing.

On the drawing, you will find the holes that will show you where to get into the ends of the elastic bands and then sew them to fix.

The last is sewn the 2 folder sides

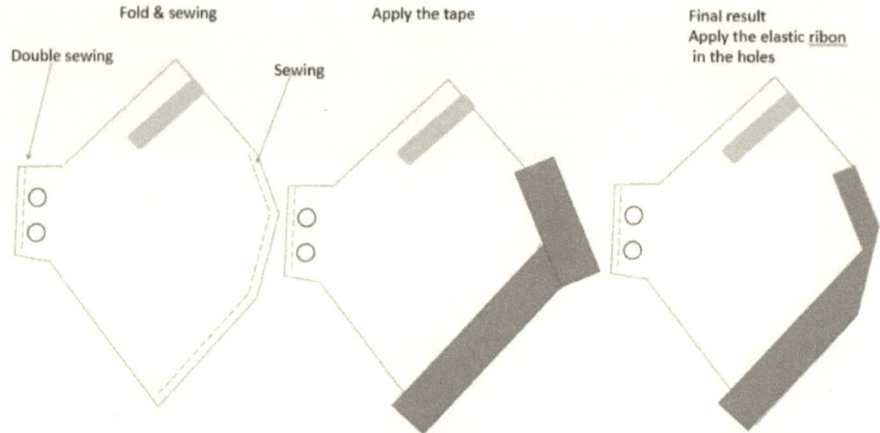

Another interesting cut pattern

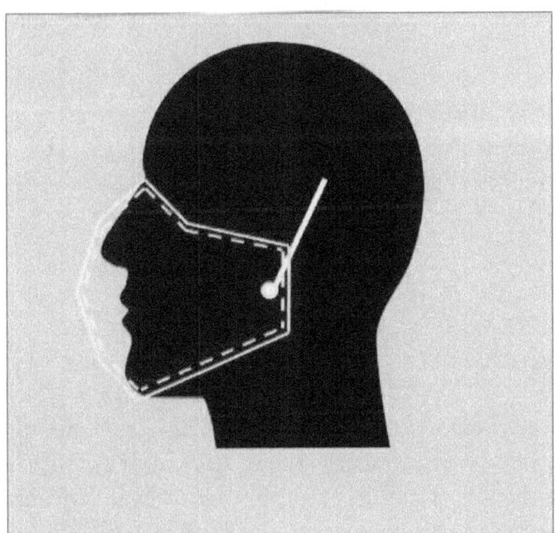

Please find another pattern that can be used with clothes and fabrics, the process is the same as previous ones.

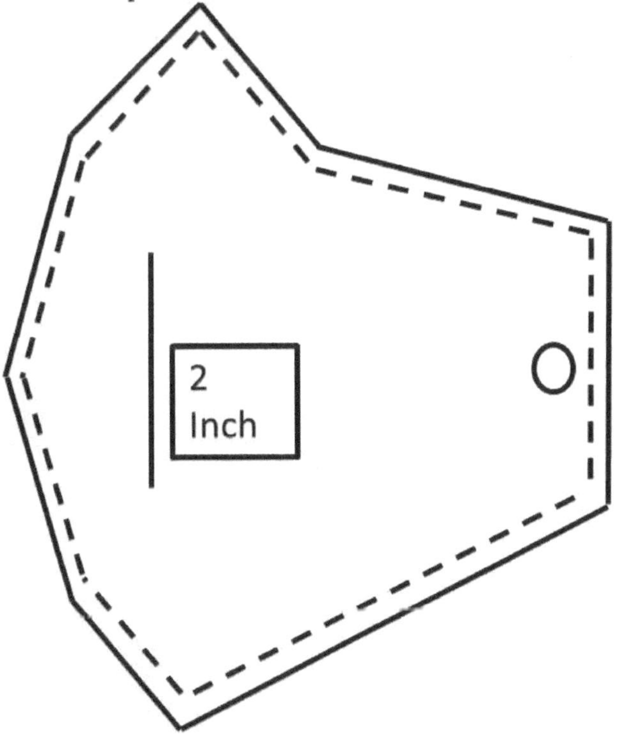

Reference and acknowledgments

Virus Image

By https://www.scientificanimations.com -
https://www.scientificanimations.com/wiki-images/, CC BY-SA 4.0,
https://commons.wikimedia.org/w/index.php? curid = 86436446

WHO: *www.Who.int*

https://www.scmp.com/news/hong-kong/health-environment/article/3050689/how-make-your-own-mask-hong-kong-scientists

(Davies, Anna & Thompson, Katy-Anne & Giri, Karthika & Kafatos, George & Walker, James & Bennett, Allan. (2013). Testing the Efficacy of Homemade Masks: Would They Protect in a Pandemic Influence ?. Disaster medicine and public health preparedness. 7.413-418.10.1017 / dmp.2013.43.)

CONCLUSION

Thank you for acquiring and reading this book to this end.

With the frequent outbreak of infectious epidemics that can be transmitted by a touch of the hand, the hand sanitizers are no longer an option but must-have equipment.

Lessons learned from epidemics such as SARS, MERS, and of late, COVID-19 proves that 'a stitch in time saves nine.' It further proves that 'to be prepared is to be forearmed.' And from time immemorial, the maxim that 'prevention is better than cure' holds supreme.

Yet, the biggest lesson that we have learned from these epidemics is that just knowing where to get hand sanitizers is insufficient. Worse of it, saving money so that you can buy the hand sanitizer during epidemics is akin to building your castle in the air.

Skills are supreme. Learning how to make your own sanitizer is what will make you sew that stitch in time, be forearmed, and ultimately prevent life-threatening epidemics. During an epidemic, the skills on how to make hand sanitizers are more important than the ready-made hand sanitizers that can easily run out of stock. Yet, these skills are more important than having loads of money to buy hand sanitizers that may not be available when you need them most.

The supremacy of skills is unquestionable. And it is for this reason that I wrote this hands-on practical guide on how to prepare your own home-made hand sanitizer. These are life-saving skills. Thousands of lives have been lost to SARS, MERS, and of late, COVID-19. Yours need not be added to this fatal statistic. And neither should be that of your loved ones. Be forearmed to fight this battle.

I am confident that the information provided in this book has enabled you to prepare your own home-made hand sanitizer. If that be the case, please encourage your loved ones, colleagues, and others to acquire a copy of this book so that they, too, may equip themselves with these life-saving skills.

Again, thank you for acquiring this book.

Good Luck!

ABOUT THE AUTHOR

Jameka Watkins is the New York Times bestselling author of The Joy of Leaving Your Sh*t All Over the Place. She is also the author of Cocktails for Drinkers, Poetry from Scratch and the novel Afloat. Her work has appeared in the Atlantic, Teen Vogue and on BBC Radio 4.